*Everyday
Aromatherapy*

Everyday Aromatherapy

Karen Philip

Introduction by Susan Fraser

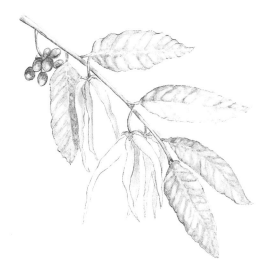

BROCKHAMPTON PRESS

This edition published 1994 by Brockhampton Press,
a member of Hodder Headline PLC Group.
Reprinted 1997.

ISBN 1 86019 011 1

Printed and bound in UAE.

Contents

Introduction

Natural healing methods should be used to treat the person as a whole and not used to isolate a part of the body or its symptoms. Essential oils are best used in this way and although it takes professional training to give a holistic treatment, the oils can be used very successfully and safely at home to alleviate stress, promote relaxation, as minor first aid (e.g. lavender on burns), and to improve general health. They can also be used in many ways around the home and for beauty care.

Essential oils are powerful substances and only a very small amount is required to bring about an effect. It is imperative for any aspect of aromatherapy that only true natural essential oils from a reputable supplier are used—a synthetic fragrance will not do. Anyone with severe medical symptoms should seek professional medical advice. If you are in any doubt regarding health, or the use of oils, contact a professional aromatherapist.

Susan Fraser, S.P.Dip.A., D.T.M., M.I.S.P.A.
Centre for Complementary Therapies, Inverness.

The History of Aromatherapy

The Egyptians were well aware of the value of essential oils and even had them imported from other countries. Surviving hieroglyphs depict high priests and alchemists blending aromatic substances to make perfumes and medicinal potions. In fact, use of aromatherapy was widespread in Egyptian pharmacology and had a great variety of practical applications. Egyptian high priests had a sophisticated knowledge of the potential action of different aromas upon the psyche and the body—they had even developed a contraceptive recipe. Kyphi, the soothing incense, was developed by the Egyptians from essential oils to allay fears and induce a sense of well being without the side-effects of alcohol or mind expanding drugs.

The Bible refers frequently to the use of essential oils for healing and religious ceremonies. The best known Biblical reference to essential oils is to be found in the tale of the three kings who travelled to bring the infant Christ the gifts of gold, frankincense and myrrh.

In the Middle Ages, monks cultivated herbs specifically to exploit their restorative properties, and the crusaders reintroduced perfumery to Europe in the 12th century. Perhaps it was no coincidence that perfumers seemed immune to the medieval scourges of cholera and other normally fatal diseases. Although in these times perfumes composed of essential oils were generally used in order to mask the unpleasant odours of seldom-washed bodies, they were also recognised for their prophylactic properties in the fight against disease.

In renaissance times, the herbal pharmacopoeia was well established and essential oils could be bought from the apothecary to treat a wide manner of ills. Scientific progress however, saw a decline in the use of essential oils which were gradually replaced with chemical substitutes which were usually cheaper and easier to mass produce. Whilst these produced reasonable perfumes, their therapeutic benefits were often inferior to those of essential oils. Furthermore, their use was frequently accompanied by unpleasant side-effects.

Aromatics Today

Whilst people may be sceptical about the power or effectiveness of essential oils, most of us practice aromatherapy unwittingly in our everyday lives. Most people would choose to plant certain flowers and plants in their gardens because of their perfume. Rose gardens are often designed to accommodate seating in order that the owners may linger to unwind in the relaxing aroma. Few cooks eschew the use of aromatic herbs, and it can be no coincidence that those herbs chosen for their fragrance and their flavour (such as ginger, rosemary and thyme) also happen to stimulate the secretion of gastric juices which aid digestion. Many automatically turn to proprietary remedies for chesty colds and coughs which contain eucalyptus, a favoured aromatherapy treatment for these complaints. For those us who like to wallow in scented baths, a glance at the ingredients of our favourite bath oil will doubtless reveal that it contains several essential oils added for their relaxing properties. Today, the use of essential oils is increasing in popularity as more and more people become increasingly aware of the side effects of many artificially manufactured drugs.

The Value of Aromatherapy

Essential oils work with the body rather than against it so that it is encouraged to heal itself and return to a state of equilibrium. Aromatherapy is also a holistic approach to health—the aromatherapist aims to treat the whole person rather than just the disease or complaint. It also has the considerable benefit of being an **enjoyable** treatment, with the added advantage that it is extremely effective in relieving stress. It has been scientifically proven that stress undermines our immune systems, and therefore our ability to resist disease. Another advantage of aromatherapy is that it provides considerable opportunity for self-help and self knowledge, invaluable weapons in the quest for health and well being. Furthermore, human beings derive enormous comfort and solace from the touch of others, a basic need for human contact inherent in us all from the moment of birth. However, many do not have the opportunity to give or receive the comfort of a hug or a cuddle when we are ill or in pain. The action of rubbing a painful or sore limb, for instance, is instinctive to everyone, which is why the use of essential oils combined with massage is so effective in relieving pain or tension.

Essential Oils

Essential oils—those odiferous 'living' substances extracted from wild or cultivated plants—are vital to aromatherapy. They bear little resemblance to the heavy oils we employ in cookery (such as olive or corn oil)—in fact, they are much lighter than water, extremely concentrated and highly flammable. The molecular structure of essential oil enables them to penetrate the skin much more readily than the more familiar domestic oils. Often known as the 'life-force' and the 'soul' of a plant, they give it its characteristic smell. A few leaves of lavender or rosemary squeezed or rubbed on the fingers, for instance, will leave microscopic particles of the essential oil of the plant on your skin which will linger for some time.

Almost all flowers, seeds, grains, barks, roots, leaves and resins contain essential oils, albeit in minute quantities. Some plants will yield more than one oil: for instance, the orange contains one oil in the skin of the fruit, another in the leaves and yet another in the flowers.

Each essential oil is credited with its own specific therapeutic properties, whilst all have antibiotic, antiseptic and anti-inflammatory properties to a greater or lesser degree, and some are believed to have anti-viral properties. Used correctly in aromatherapy, these oils seem to have further positive effects. It would appear that they boost the immune system thereby improving the body's chances of invading microbes, and promote healing by stimulating cell-regrowth. Certain oils may improve circulation, whilst others have an analgesic effect, or the ability to relieve fluid retention, in fact a wide variety of complaints.

The Ancient Egyptians used essential oils in embalming or mummification processes because they were well aware of their ability to thwart the proliferation of the microbes which cause decomposition of flesh. Hippocrates encouraged the townspeople of Athens to burn aromatic plants in the streets in order to prevent the spread of plague. In fact, as late as the last war, maternity wards were fumigated and surgical instruments sterilised in dilutions of essential oils such as clove, lemon, thyme, and chamomile.

It would seem that not only do such naturally-derived antibiotics kill harmful microbes, they also encourage the immune system to resist further infection. This is worth taking into consideration, as today's manufactured antibiotics tend to destroy not only harmful bacteria but also those beneficial bacteria which live in the alimentary canal. Essential oils, then, would seem to be an extremely powerful ally in the fight against disease.

Since Egyptian times, essential oils have been prized for their anti-inflammatory properties, but used correctly have none of the side effects of modern anti-inflammatory drugs such as steroids.

Essential Oils—
The Main Extraction Techniques

Extraction techniques vary according to where in the plant the oil is situated. For example, in the Labitiae family of plants (which includes peppermint and lavender) the essential oil glands are readily accessible on the outside of the leaves. In their case, the choice of extraction method is distillation. This involves packing fresh or dried flowers tightly into a still and then passing steam through it. During this process, the glands burst and the oil evaporates into steam. When cooled, the essential oils will separate from the water. In plants such as tea tree or myrtle, the glands are in a less accessible position and the leaves may require bruising before distillation.

Plants such as the citrus varieties may lend themselves to the simplest method of extraction which is expression. This can be done either by hand or machine, and involves squeezing or scraping the peels and rinds of the fruits. The oil is collected into a sponge which is simply squeezed when saturated.

Another fairly simple method of extraction is maceration, in which flowers are soaked in hot oil until their cells burst, releasing the essential oil into the base oil. The oil is then purified and the aromatic substances extracted by a process known as defleurage. A variation of this technique is enfleurage. Top-quality undamaged flowers are crushed between trays smeared with fat until the fat has absorbed the perfume. This is followed by a defleurage technique similar to that already mentioned. Essential oils obtained in this way tend to be of a superior quality compared to those obtained by distillation, and are accordingly more expensive.

In the case of the most delicate flowers the choice of extraction method is solvent extraction. Tonnes of fresh flowers are centrifuged with a solvent until the oils and waxes have separated from the waste material and solvent. The oils and waxes are then vacuum distilled at a low temperature in order to separate them.

Finally, a word about purchasing essential oils. Always choose a reputable dealer and avoid anything labelled 'aromatherapy' as it is unlikely to contain pure essences. They will probably have been bulked out with a high percentage of mineral or vegetable oil. (Mineral oil is useless for aromatherapy as its molecules are too large to penetrate the skin.) Many essential oils are expensive due to complicated extraction procedures and the requirement of large quantities of the raw material. For instance, it takes 2000 kg of jasmine to produce 1kg of essential oil. However, it may be that some dealers charge higher prices than necessary because they buy oil in small quantities, so it pays to shop around.

Jasmine

Base Oils

Because essential oils are extremely concentrated and also because of their tendency to evaporate rapidly, they need to be diluted with carrier or base oils. Generally it is not advised that essential oils should be applied undiluted to the skin, although there are one or two specific exceptions. It is very important to use a high quality base oil, as oils such as baby or mineral oil have very poor penetrating qualities which will hamper the passage of the essential oil through the skin. Indeed, it would be better to use a good quality vegetable or nut oil for babies in preference to proprietary baby oils as the vegetable oil is more easily absorbed and contains more nutrients!

Pure essential oils should retain their potency for one to two years, but once diluted in a base oil will only last for three months or so. They should also be stored at a fairly constant room temperature in amber glass bottles as they will deteriorate quickly when subjected to extremes of light and temperature. For massage oils, it is best to make up a very small quantity of essential oil in base oil for each application because of its poor keeping qualities.

Below is a very rough guide to the dilution of essential oils. However, you will find many variations and differing opinions on this depending on the preference of individual therapists, and their recipes will differ accordingly.

Base or Carrier Oil	Essential Oil
100 ml	20–60 drops
25 ml	7–25 drops
1 teaspoon (5 ml)	3–5 drops

Although the choice of base oil is largely a matter of personal preference, it is useful to note that many vegetable oils possess therapeutic properties of their own. Any of sweet almond, soya bean, sunflower, jojoba, olive, grapeseed, hazelnut, avocado, corn or safflower will provide a suitable base for essential oils although these should preferably be of the cold-pressed variety which have higher nutrient levels.

Treatment Techniques

Blending essential oils:

Essences can be blended to treat specific ailments, and some aromatherapy books contain precise recipes for blends. When two or more essential oils are working together in harmony, this is known as a synergistic blend. Obviously, it takes many years of experience to know which combinations of plant essences will work most effectively together, but as a rough guide, oils extracted from plants of the same botanical family will usually blend and work well together, although it is by no means necessary to stick rigidly to this rule as other combinations may be just as successful. Really, a number of factors need to be taken into account when preparing a blend of oils for a patient, such as the nature of his/her complaint, his personality or frame of mind. For home use, it is not usually beneficial to blend more than three oils for any one preparation.

Massage:

Massage is perhaps the most important aromatherapy technique and the one favoured by most trained aromatherapists. An aromatherapist will 'design' an individual whole body massage based on an accurate history taken from the patient and much experience in the use of essential oils. The oils will be chosen specifically to match the temperament of the patient and also to deal with any particular medical or emotional problems which may be troubling him or her.

Although there is no substitute for a long soothing aromatherapy massage given by an expert, the techniques are not difficult to learn and can be carried out satisfactorily at home.

Hair treatments/scalp tonics:

Many hair conditions such as dryness/excessive grease, or dandruff will respond to aromatherapy using specific recipes of essential oils diluted in a nourishing base oil. For instance, 60 drops of an essential oil diluted in 100 mls of base oil (such as olive or sweet almond) will make a wonderful conditioning treatment. Simply rub the oils thoroughly into the scalp, then wrap the hair in warm towels and allow the oil to penetrate the hair and the scalp for an hour or two. The choice of oil depends of course upon the desired effect: chamomile and rosemary, for instance will condition and promote healthy hair growth, bergamot and tea tree are helpful in dandruff control whilst lavender has repellent qualities which will deter lice and fleas.

Face creams, oils, lotions and treatments for skin problems:

For the face, essential oils should be mixed with base oils in much the same way as for massage, the main difference being that more nourishing oils such as apricot kernel and avocado should be used in preference to ordinary vegetable oils. (It should be noted that avocado is a fairly heavy oil and its use is best reserved for dry skin.) Essential oils can also be added to a non-perfumed cold cream or lotion and used for problem complexions.

Most essential oils have antiseptic properties and can be used to treat infective skin conditions. Certain oils (such as rose and neroli) are anti-inflammatory and have a soothing effect, whereas sandalwood is useful in the treatment of superficial broken veins. Rose and neroli are also excellent for care of mature skins. For dry cracked skin, the addition of wheatgerm and avocado (with their high vitamin E content) oil to preparations will relieve the condition. In general, aromatherapy can improve the skin by encouraging toxin removal, stimulating cell growth and renewal and improving circulation. A gentle circular massage with the tips of the fingers should be used on the face, and special care must be taken not to stretch or drag the delicate skin around the eye area.

Flower waters:

Flower waters constitute a refreshing and soothing aid in the treatment and prevention of skin conditions such as eczema and acne, and can be easily prepared at home. Simply add around 20 drops of essential oil to an amber glass bottle containing 100 mls of spring water, then leave it to stand in a dark place for a few days. Filter the water through some coffee or similar filter paper, then apply to the skin as required using a cotton wool pad.

Compresses:

Compresses are effective in the treatment of a variety of muscular and rheumatic aches and pains as well as bruises and headaches.

To prepare a compress, add 5 drops of essential oil to a small bowl of water. Soak a piece of flannel or sheeting of other absorbent material in the solution. Squeeze out excess moisture (although the compress should remain fairly wet) and secure in position with a bandage or cling film. For acute pain, the compress should be renewed when it has reached blood temperature, otherwise it should be left in position for a minimum of two hours and preferably overnight. Generally speaking, cold water should be used wherever fever or acute pain or hot swelling require treatment, whereas the water should be hot if the pain is chronic.

N.B. If fever is present, the compress should be changed frequently.

Bathing and showering:

Add a few drops (5-10) of essential oil to the bath water after the water has been drawn, then close the door to retain the aromatic vapours. The choice of oils is entirely up to the individual, depending on the desired effect, although those with sensitive skins are advised to have the oils ready diluted in a base oil prior to bathing. Bathing in essential oils can stimulate and revive or relax and sedate depending on the oils selected: rosemary and pine can have a soothing effect on tired or aching limbs, chamomile and lavender are popular for relieving insomnia and anxiety etc. A similar effect (although obviously not quite as relaxing) can be achieved whilst showering by soaking a wet sponge in essential oil mix, then rubbing it over the body under the warm spray.

Essential oils can damage the surface of many modern baths if not added to a carrier.

Sitz bath:

A sitz bath in the appropriate essential oil can bring enormous relief in conditions such as haemorrhoids, thrush and cystitis.

Foot bath:

Tired, swollen feet can be refreshed by bathing in a basin of hot water containing 4-5 drops of lavender, peppermint, rosemary or thyme.

Hands:

Dry, chapped hands may be soothed by soaking in a bowl of warm water containing a few drops of essential oil such as patchouli or rose.

Mouthwash and gargles:

Used strictly in the correct dilutions, essential oils provide a natural, gentle way to help clear up mouth ulcers, oral thrush and infected gums, but it cannot be stressed too much that essential oils should NEVER be swallowed.

Inhalation:

Place a few drops of an essential oil such as thyme or peppermint in a basin of hot, steaming water then drape a towel over the head and bowl and breathe deeply for a minute or two. Repeat several times, for as long as the water remains hot. Steam inhalation with essential oils constitutes a wonderful, time-honoured way of alleviating the symptoms of colds and flu, and can also be beneficial to greasy skins. Steam inhalations should, however, be avoided by asthmatics unless under direction from a medical practitioner, as the steam can occasionally irritate the lungs.

Neat application and internal use:

Generally, the application of undiluted essential oils directly to the skin should be avoided as many are highly irritant. However, there are one or two exceptions which have been safely applied to the skin undiluted for centuries. These include lemon oil, which can be applied neat to warts (Vaseline can be applied around the wart to protect the surrounding skin); lavender, which can be safely applied directly to burns, cuts, bites and stings; and tea tree, which may be dabbed on spots. Any other oils must be used in dilution unless under careful direction from a trained aromatherapist.

Many essential oils are highly toxic when taken orally and there are NO CIRCUMSTANCES in which they may safely be taken at home in this way.

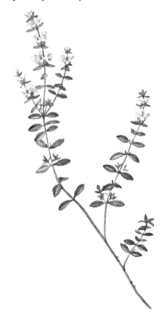

Thyme (Sweet)

Essential Oils Around the Home

There are a variety of ways in which your home can be enhanced by the use of essential oils. Fragrances, pomanders, ring burners and diffusers can all be used in conjunction with essential oils to impart a wonderful scent to a room. (Essential oils should be put into water and vapourized and not burned as they are inflammable. Follow the instructions on ring burners carefully and never put essential oils directly onto a hot light bulb.) Most essential oils also have anti-microbial properties which make them extremely useful when the occupants of the room are suffering from colds and flu. Oils such as myrtle and eucalyptus also seem to have a soothing effect on coughs and can be used in the bedroom where they will release their aroma throughout the night. Fragrancers, pomanders, and ring burners can all be purchased quite cheaply from shops and indeed make very welcome gifts, but the same effect can be achieved by adding a few drops of essential oil in a bowl of water and placing it on a radiator. In case of colds or flu, a bowl of water is actually preferable as it has a humidifying effect on the air.

Three or 4 four drops of an appropriate essential oil such as eucalyptus sprinkled on a handkerchief can be inhaled periodically to alleviate the worst symptoms of colds. Similarly, 2-3 drops of a relaxing essential oil on the pillow at night can help to cure insomnia.

Essential Oils— How They Work

Inhalation, application and bathing are the three main methods used to encourage the entry of essential oils into the body. When inhaled, the extremely volatile oils may enter via the olfactory system, and permeation of the skin occurs when they are diluted and applied externally. By bathing in essential oils, we can inhale and absorb the oils through the skin simultaneously.

Little is known about how essential oils actually affect the mind and the body, although research is currently ongoing in the USA and the UK. However, the effectiveness of aromatherapy has been supported by recent research in central Europe, the USA, the UK and Australia. It appears that most essential oils are antiseptic and bactericidal to greater or lesser degrees, whilst some even seem to be effective in fighting viral infections.

On inhalation, essential oil molecules are received by receptor cells in the lining of the nose, which will transmit signals to the brain. Electrochemical messages received by the olfactory centre in the brain then stimulate the release of powerful neurochemicals into the blood which will then be transported around the body. Molecules inhaled into the lungs may pass into the bloodstream and be disseminated in the same way.

When rubbed or massaged into the skin, essential oils will permeate the pores and hair follicles. From here, they can readily pass into the tiny blood vessels (known as capillaries) by virtue of their molecular structure, and then travel around the body.

Once absorbed, the action of the oil depends upon its chemical constituents. Most essential oils are high in alcohols and esters, although a few contain a high concentration of phenols, aldehydes and ketones. The latter are powerful chemicals and their use should be avoided by all save the skilled professional.

Essential Oils to be Avoided for Home Use

You may find that your professional aromatherapist will use some of the following oils, but these are generally unsafe for use by the lay person.

Generally	*During Pregnancy*	*Prior to Exposure to Sun*
Aniseed	Basil	Bergamot
Cinnamon Bark	Cedarwood	Lemon
Cinnamon Leaf	Clary Sage	Mandarin
Clove Bud	Fennel	Orange
Clove Leaf	Juniper	
Clove Stem	Marjoram	
Fennel (Bitter)	Myrrh	
Pine	Rosemary	
	Sage	
	Thyme	

Hypertension (High Blood Pressure)
Sage
Thyme

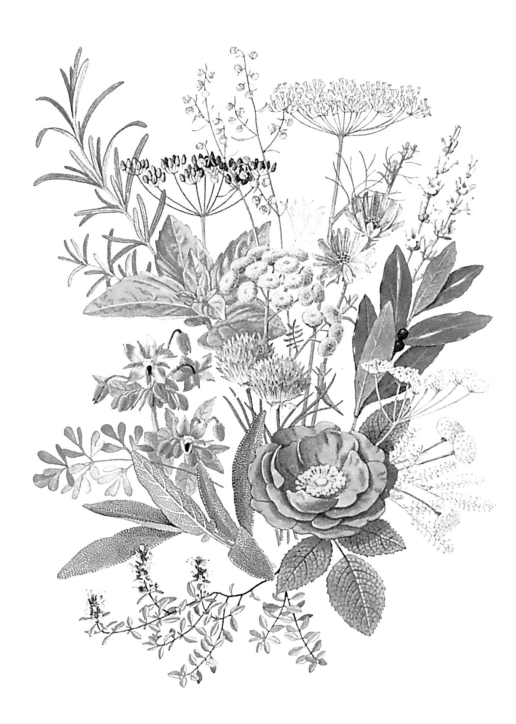

The Essential Oils A–Z

The following section is by no means an exhaustive one, but aims to include the most popular oils readily available today. Similarly, whilst therapeutic uses have been suggested, aromatherapists will differ in the choice of oils for particular complaints, just as a general practitioner may prescribe one remedy for a specific complaint, whereas his partner in the same practice may favour another treatment for the same complaint.

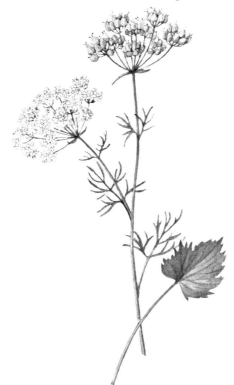

Aniseed

Aniseed
(Pimpinella anisum)

FAMILY: Apiacea (*Umbelliferae*)

DERIVATION: By steam distillation from the seed of the plant.

ORIGINS/HISTORY: Native to Greece and Egypt, but also widely grown in India and China, Mexico and Spain. The Romans used aniseed as a breath sweetener, an aphrodisiac, and as a stimulant to breast milk production. Records exist of aniseed cultivation in European herb gardens as far back as the 14th century.

THERAPEUTIC PROPERTIES/APPLICATIONS: Aniseed seems to have a carminative (flatulence expelling) effect on the alimentary canal and is therefore useful in the treatment of infantile colic, flatulence and indigestion.

The anti-spasmodic property of aniseed can also be effective against period pains.

Aniseed seems to stimulate lactation post-natally and is used in lozenges and cough sweets for its decongestant effect. Its anti-parasitic effect makes it useful in the treatment of lice and scabies.

Aniseed has a strong antiseptic effect.

OTHER USES: Provides the taste in cough lozenges. Can be used for cooking with and also of use in the manufacture of certain alcoholic drinks, such as Pernod.

SAFETY PRECAUTIONS/CONTRAINDICATIONS: Can be irritant to sensitive skins. Can be narcotic in large doses and should only be used in moderation.

ANISEED OIL MUST BE USED BY A TRAINED AROMATHERAPIST AND IS UNSAFE FOR HOME USE.

Basil
(Omicum basilicum)

FAMILY: Lamiaceae (*Labitiae*)

DERIVATION: By steam distillation from the whole plant.

ORIGINS/HISTORY: Basil is originally a native of Africa and the Seychelles, but is now grown and used widely throughout Europe. Greek nobles bathed in essential oil of basil and the ancient Egyptians mixed it with myrrh and incense for use in their embalming processes. Basil is sacred to the Gods Krishna and Vishnu in India, where it is believed to protect the soul from evil. Essential oil of basil is still widely used in Eastern medicine today. In this country, the oil was mainly used to scent snuff.

THERAPEUTIC APPLICATIONS/PROPERTIES: Basil is valued for its uplifting effects—it alleviates fatigue and depression and has a general tonic effect. It is also credited with being able to clear the head and aid concentration.
Basil can be effective in treating respiratory infections such as colds, bronchitis, asthma and sinusitis. It can also alleviate the symptoms of fever, gout and indigestion. It seems to be equally effective in baths, inhalation and massage, and its strongly antiseptic effect makes it a good choice for soothing skin abrasions and assisting the healing process. It also has insect repellent qualities. As a digestive aid, basil's anti-spasmodic effect has made it a favoured herb in cookery throughout the ages.

SAFETY PRECAUTIONS/CONTRAINDICATIONS: Basil should be avoided during pregnancy. Can also have a depressant effect, so it should be used in moderation. Relatively non-toxic, but should be well diluted to avoid possible skin irritation.

Bay
(Laurus nobilis)

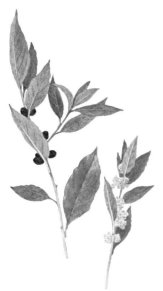

FAMILY: Lauraceae

DERIVATION: Extracted by steam distillation from dried leaves and berries.

ORIGINS / HISTORY: Widely cultivated throughout the warmer countries of the world, but native to the Mediterranean. In classical mythology, the Bay Tree was sacred to Apollo, the god of medicine, and Roman Emperors sported sprigs of *laurus nobilis* to signify victory, wealth and learning and to protect them from evil spirits. The Romans burnt bay in public places during outbreaks of plague in order to thwart the spread of the disease. Like the Romans, medieval women used talismans of bay to ward off the 'evil eye'. Ancient Greeks would chew on bay leaves to freshen the breath after banquets.

THERAPEUTIC APPLICATIONS / PROPERTIES: Both *laurus nobilis* and its West Indian cousin *pimenta racemosa* are valuable in the treatment of colds, flu and bronchitis. As discovered by the ancients, it also promotes digestion, and combats dyspepsia and flatulence. The West Indian oil is favoured in the treatment of rheumatic pain because of its anti-inflammatory properties and is widely used as a general tonic. Both can be used in inhalation, baths and massage.

OTHER USES: Bay is widely used by perfumers because of its uplifting effect.

SAFETY PRECAUTIONS / CONTRAINDICATIONS: Avoid application to sensitive skins.

Benzoin

(Styrax benzoin)

FAMILY: Styracaceae

DERIVATION: The gum is taken from the bark of the tree.

ORIGINS / HISTORY: For thousands of years, benzoin has been used in the East both as a medicine and an incense, and was believed to have the power to keep evil spirits at bay. Chinese herbalists valued it as an aid to digestion and as a urinary antiseptic. In the west, it has been used for centuries in the form of Friar's Balsam in the treatment of respiratory infections.

THERAPEUTIC APPLICATIONS / PROPERTIES: For skin complaints, benzoin is indicated in the treatment of chapped, inflamed or irritated skin. Its antiseptic properties make it a popular choice for urinary, respiratory and throat infections. Benzoin also has uplifting qualities which can relieve stress and nervous tension when used in a massage oil. As an expectorant, many therapists recommend a few drops of benzoin in a pint of hot water as an inhalation.

OTHER USES: Dentists often use compound tincture of benzoin (Friar's Balsam) to treat inflamed gums, and essential oil of benzoin is a popular fragrance ingredient in the production of perfumes, soaps and toiletries.

SAFETY PRECAUTIONS / CONTRAINDICATIONS: Compound tincture of benzoin (which contains other substances including aloe, Tolu balsam and storax) occasionally causes sensitivity, but benzoin itself is generally non-toxic and non-irritant to most individuals.

Bergamot
(Citrus bergamia)

FAMILY: Rutaceae

DERIVATION: The oil is extracted by cold expression of the peel of the fruit.

ORIGINS/HISTORY: Originally a native of Asia, although it was discovered by Columbus in the Canary Islands at the time of his great voyages. It is named after the city of Bergamot in Northern Italy, where Italians first traded in the oil. Bergamot oil has been used in Italian folk medicine for centuries, mainly for the treatment of fever and intestinal parasites.

THERAPEUTIC APPLICATIONS/PROPERTIES: Recent research carried out in Italy indicates a wide variety of therapeutic applications for Bergamot, including urinary tract and respiratory infections. Its strong antiseptic effect makes it a good choice for the treatment of skin, throat and mouth infections. In particular skin conditions such as psoriasis, acne and ulcers will often respond to bergamot, especially where stress and depression may have played a part in lowering resistance to infection. When combined with eucalyptus, its soothing effect will afford relief to sufferers of cold sores and shingles. Insomnia and depression can be alleviated by the uplifting and refreshing nature of this oil.

OTHER USES: A popular ingredient in perfumes and cosmetics, bergamot is widely employed as a food ingredient. Its heady aroma gives Earl Grey tea its unique quality.

SAFETY PRECAUTIONS/CONTRAINDICATIONS: Bergamot can irritate the skin if used in concentrations in excess of one per cent. It is phototoxic and should not be used in home-made suntan oil.

Cajeput
(Melaleuca cajeputi)

FAMILY: Myrtaceae

DERIVATION: The essential oil is obtained from the leaves and twigs by steam distillation.

ORIGINS/HISTORY: Cajeput grows wild in Indonesia, Malaysia, the Philippines, Java, Vietnam, Australia and South East Asia. The plant is much valued in Eastern herbal medicine, having a wide variety of applications as a treatment for colds, sore throats, headaches, muscle fatigue and strain, rheumatism and toothache. The Western herbal tradition has used the oil to treat bronchitis and laryngitis, urinary tract infections, bronchitis and to rid sufferers of some intestinal parasites.

THERAPEUTIC APPLICATIONS/PROPERTIES: In addition to the above, therapists have found cajeput helpful for relief of a wide variety of complaints. Used in baths, diffusers, inhalation and massage, cajeput can bring relief from asthma, bronchitis, sinusitis and throat infections. Occasionally it has been used to treat diarrhoea and indigestion.

OTHER USES: Used in many dental formulations, and a popular ingredient in detergents, perfumes and soaps.

SAFETY PRECAUTIONS/CONTRAINDICATIONS: May be irritant to the skin if used in high concentrations.

Cedarwood

(Juniperus virginiana)

FAMILY: Cupressaceae

DERIVATION: Extracted from waste woods by steam distillation.

ORIGINS/HISTORY: A native of North America, where the indigenous Indians valued it in the treatment of catarrhal infections. Another species (*Cedrus atlantica*) was used by the Egyptians for embalming, and Tibetans frequently used it as an incense. In the 19th century, the oil was popular for scenting handkerchiefs and as a fragrance ingredient in soap.

THERAPEUTIC APPLICATIONS/PROPERTIES: Cedarwood seems to be beneficial in skin and scalp conditions such as alopecia, acne, dandruff and eczema. It also helps the body to fight respiratory infections and problems and has a mild diuretic effect which can be useful in the treatment of urinary tract infections. Cedarwood has been credited with aphrodisiac qualities.

OTHER USES: Cedarwood is extremely useful as a household insect repellent, and is popular in the manufacture of perfumes, particularly in masculine scents.

SAFETY PRECAUTIONS/CONTRAINDICATIONS: High concentrations may irritate the skin, and on NO ACCOUNT must cedarwood be used during pregnancy as it is a powerful abortifacient.

Chamomile (Roman)
(Anthemus nobilis)

FAMILY: Asteraceae

DERIVATION: The oil is extracted from flower heads by steam distillation.

ORIGINS/HISTORY: Native to Europe and north-west Asia, chamomile has a long-standing reputation in treatment of conditions in which stress and tension are contributory factors.

THERAPEUTIC APPLICATIONS/PROPERTIES: There are several varieties, but Roman Chamomile is the essential oil of choice for home use. It is used by therapists to treat many skin complaints and promotes the healing of burns, cuts, bites and inflammations. It is also effective in allergic conditions and can have a beneficial effect

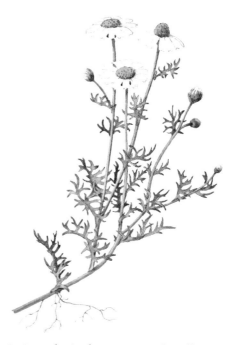

on menstrual problems when used regularly in the bath. It seems to be effective in reducing stress and anxiety and problems such as headache, migraine and insomnia. As an analgesic, it is used in the treatment of earache, toothache, neuralgia and abscesses, and is popular for treating childhood illnesses.

OTHER USES: Chamomile is often used in proprietary antiseptic ointments, shampoos and toiletries and as a fragrance in high-class perfumes.

SAFETY PRECAUTIONS/CONTRAINDICATIONS: Chamomile is generally non-toxic and non-irritant, but may cause dermatitis in very sensitive individuals.

Cinnamon
(Cinnamomum zeylanicum)

FAMILY: Lauraceae

DERIVATION: By steam or water distillation from the twigs and leaves or from the dried inner bark.

Origins / History: Cinnamon originally comes from Sri Lanka, but also grows abundantly in Brazil, Mauritius, India and Madagascar. Cinnamon has been used in the East for thousands of years in the treatment of a wide variety of illnesses including colds and flu, digestive and menstrual problems. It is said to have been given to King Solomon by the Queen of Sheba, and the legendary phoenix used it in the construction of its pyre.

THERAPEUTIC APPLICATIONS / PROPERTIES: This oil possesses a warm, spicy aroma and has been favoured in the treatment of nausea, dyspepsia, flatulence and other digestive disturbances. Its warm, soothing qualities can be beneficial to rheumatism when used in massage oil on the affected parts. These soothing, relaxing qualities also impart a strong stress-relieving effect.

OTHER USES: Cinnamon oil is used extensively in cookery and as a flavouring agent for commercially prepared foodstuffs, including coca-cola. It is also a popular ingredient for cough medicines, lozenges and dental preparations.

SAFETY PRECAUTIONS / CONTRAINDICATIONS: Cinnamon can be irritant to the mucous membranes in very large doses. That oil which is distilled from the bark is especially irritant to both skin and mucous membranes and should never be directly applied.

> CINNAMON OIL MUST BE USED BY A TRAINED AROMATHERAPIST AND IS UNSAFE
> FOR HOME USE.

Clary Sage
(*Salvia sclarea*)

FAMILY: Lamiaceae (*Labiatae*)

DERIVATION: The essential oil is obtained by steam distillation from the leaves and the flowers.

ORIGINS/HISTORY: Clary sage was originally a native of Syria and was first introduced to Britain in 1562. It is now cultivated worldwide. Employed in ancient and medieval times, sage seems to have fallen into disuse for a time, although its use was revived towards the end of the 19th century. In the middle ages particularly, it was used for a variety of ailments including kidney problems, menstrual and uterine disorders, for skin ulcers and as an uplifting tonic. It was a popular perfume fixative, especially in France.

THERAPEUTIC APPLICATIONS/PROPERTIES: Clary sage is possessed of antispasmodic, anti-depressant, balsamic, carminative, tonic, aperitive, astringent, anti-inflammatory, bactericidal and antiseptic qualities. It is valuable in stress related conditions, and has an anti-hypertensive effect. A thick mucilage can be made from the seeds, which was traditionally used for removing particles of dust from the eyes. Clary sage is also indicated in the treatment of colds and throat infections. It is also good for regulating oily skin and menstrual problems.

OTHER USES: Used in the production of Muscatel wines. Fixative and fragrance element of perfumes, soaps, toiletries and household cleaners.

SAFETY PRECAUTIONS/CONTRAINDICATIONS: To be avoided during pregnancy. Also to be avoided in conjunction with alcohol consumption. However, in general, clary sage has very low toxicity levels and is therefore preferable to garden sage for use in aromatherapy.

Clove
(Eugenia aromatica)

FAMILY: Myrtaceae

DERIVATION: Cloves are the unopened buds of the tree, and oil is obtained by water distillation from the buds or leaves, or by steam distillation from the stems.

ORIGINS / HISTORY: Originally native to Indonesia, the clove tree is now grown throughout the world. In the Han dynasty of China, envoys to the court of the Emperor were obliged to freshen their breath with oil of cloves before the Emperor would grant them an audience. In Chinese medicine, clove has been used for centuries to relieve diarrhoea, hernia, halitosis and bronchitis. Victorian gentlemen would attempt to mask the foul stench of the streets by covering their noses with handkerchiefs scented with clove oil.

THERAPEUTIC APPLICATIONS / PROPERTIES: Clove is a useful anti-emetic and should also be used for dyspepsia. It has a powerful antiseptic and a mild analgesic action which make it popular in the relief of gum infections and aching teeth. Its expectorant effect is valuable in the treatment of bronchitis and catarrh. It is widely used as an antihistamine, and an anti-rheumatic and to treat skin conditions such as scabies and athlete's foot. It is also indicated in cuts and wounds, bruises and sprains, colds and flu.

OTHER USES: Favoured as a flavouring and an antiseptic in toothpastes and other dental preparations. A flavouring in the food industry.

SAFETY PRECAUTIONS / CONTRAINDICATIONS: Can cause mucous membrane irritation, therefore best used in small doses.

CLOVE OIL CAN BE DANGEROUS AND IS BEST USED ONLY BY A TRAINED AROMATHERAPIST.

Cypress
(Cupressus sempervirens)

FAMILY: Cupressaceae

DERIVATION: The oil is extracted mainly by steam distillation from the twigs and needles of the tree, although it can be extracted from the cones.

ORIGINS/HISTORY: Cypress was originally native to the Eastern Mediterranean countries, but now grows wild throughout many parts of Europe. Cypress was sacred to the ancient Greeks as the branches were believed to represent the gods of the underworld. It was thought that the branches could ease a person's passage into the underworld if laid across his grave. It is still used today by Tibetans in incense form for purification.

THERAPEUTIC APPLICATIONS/PROPERTIES: Cypress is thought to be beneficial to the urinary system and seems to help in conditions involving a loss of fluid. These include excessive perspiration, diarrhoea and menorrhagia. Used in the bath, cypress brings great relief to tired aching legs and feet. On the skin, or in a massage oil, its antiseptic and astringent actions can have a balancing effect on oily skin and provide an aid to healing. Cypress is often used by therapists to reduce swellings and nasal congestion, and it is useful in the treatment of colds and flu.

OTHER USES: Insect repellent. A fragrance ingredient in aftershaves and colognes.

SAFETY PRECAUTIONS/CONTRAINDICATIONS: Not to be used by those suffering from hypertension, otherwise non-irritant and non-toxic.

Eucalyptus
(Eucalyptus globulus var. globulus)

FAMILY: Myrtaceae

DERIVATION: The oil is obtained by steam distillation from the leaves and young twigs.

ORIGINS/HISTORY: Eucalyptus is indigenous to Australia and Tasmania, but has been successfully introduced to Europe, Algeria, Egypt, Tahiti, South Africa and India. The German botanist and explorer, Baron Ferdinand von Mueller, was the first person to publicise the medicinal properties of Eucalyptus. Those regions of Algeria which were planted with Eucalyptus experienced a marked reduction in the incidence of fever, and in Sicily the tree was planted extensively as a malaria preventative.

THERAPEUTIC APPLICATIONS/PROPERTIES: Eucalyptus is a strongly aromatic plant, and its oil has powerful disinfectant, stimulant, antiseptic and healing properties. It is especially popular in the treatment of respiratory complaints, such as croup and bronchitis. Parasitic skin conditions such as ringworm are often treated with Eucalyptus, as are insect bites. Its analgesic properties are often used to ease the discomfort of shingles, chicken pox and herpes, and it can have a marked effect in the reduction of fever. Therapists often use eucalyptus to soothe the pain of muscular aches and sprains.

OTHER USES: An ingredient of many pharmaceutical products: cough medicines, ointments, liniments and toothpaste. Not often used in perfumes, but often added to household cleaners, soaps and toiletries.

SAFETY PRECAUTIONS/CONTRAINDICATIONS: When diluted, eucalyptus is safe to use externally, but can be fatal if taken internally.

Fennel (Sweet)
(Foeniculum vulgare)

FAMILY: Apiaceae (*Umbelliferae*)

DERIVATION: The oil is derived from the seeds of the plant by steam distillation.

ORIGINS/HISTORY: Fennel grows wild in most parts of temperate Europe, but originally came from the shores of the Mediterranean. It was well known to the Romans—Roman soldiers frequently chewed fennel seeds on the march when meals were unavailable. Fennel was often mentioned in Anglo-Saxon cookery and medical recipes prior to the Norman conquest. Mention of fennel is also made in an ancient record of Spanish agriculture dated AD 961. In medieval times, it was hung outside cottages to keep evil spirits at bay.

THERAPEUTIC APPLICATIONS/PROPERTIES: Fennel has properties similar to those of aniseed, so that it is frequently used to treat colic and flatulence. It is also a mild natural laxative. It is credited with an action similar to oestrogen and is thought to stimulate milk production in nursing mothers. This action also indicates fennel in the treatment of menopausal symptoms. As a mild diuretic, it slows the build up of toxic waste which is a causative factor in gout and liver problems. Fennel is also suitable for children's complaints.

OTHER USES: Extensively used in pharmaceutical preparations—especially laxative and carminative preparations. A fragrance ingredient of toiletries, household cleaners, soaps and perfumes.

SAFETY PRECAUTIONS/CONTRAINDICATIONS: Avoid use on sensitive skin, or prior to exposure to sun. Should not be used by epileptics or pregnant women.

BITTER FENNEL OIL CAN BE DANGEROUS AND IS BEST USED ONLY BY A TRAINED AROMATHERAPIST.

Frankincense
(Boswellia carteri)

FAMILY: Burseraceae

DERIVATION: The oil is derived by steam distillation from the oleo gum resin.

ORIGINS / HISTORY: Frankincense is a native of the Red Sea region and Somalia. Historically used as a stimulant although it is rarely taken internally today. The ancient Egyptians used it as a rejuvenating facial preparation, and in Roman times, Pliny recommended it as an antidote to hemlock. The Romans also valued it as a religious and ceremonial oil. In the tenth century, the Arab physician Avicenna recommended it in the treatment of tumours, ulcers, vomiting dysentery and fevers. It was used until very recently in China for leprosy, and is still used today throughout the world as a holy and ceremonial incense.

THERAPEUTIC APPLICATIONS / PROPERTIES: The inhalation of Frankincense is used to relieve the symptoms of bronchitis and laryngitis, and its warm, soothing effect is useful in the treatment of asthma, attacks of which may be brought on by anxiety or emotional stress. It is also indicated in urinary tract problems such as cystitis and is sometimes used as a uterine tonic. Its healing properties have long been valued in the treatment of wounds, and it is often used in skin preparations for mature skins. It has an extremely relaxing aroma and is ideal in the bath for soothing away the day's stress.

OTHER USES: Used as a fragrance ingredient in a wide variety of perfumes. Occasionally added to pharmaceutical liniments and pastilles.

SAFETY PRECAUTIONS / CONTRAINDICATIONS: None.

Geranium

(Pelargonium graveolens)

FAMILY: Geraniaceae

DERIVATION: Obtained by steam distillation from the leaves, and also the flowers and stalks.

ORIGINS / HISTORY: Geranium has been used in herbal medicine since antiquity.

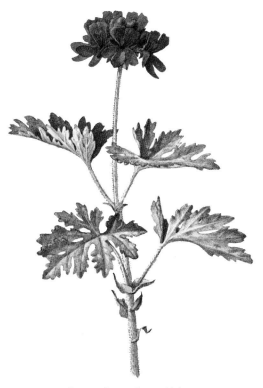

THERAPEUTIC APPLICATIONS / PROPERTIES: Geranium is an excellent 'all-round' oil, with a wide range of uses, particularly for menopausal problems and pre-menstrual tension. Its diuretic quality makes it a wise choice for fluid retention, and cellulitis and mastitis often respond well to it. For skin conditions and emotional disorders, it is a popular choice in the bath and in massage oil. Serious skin conditions often respond to its antiseptic and anti-fungal qualities.

OTHER USES: Used extensively as a fragrance in perfumery and a wide variety of cosmetics and toiletries. Also used as flavouring in the food industry.

SAFETY PRECAUTIONS / CONTRAINDICATIONS: Generally non-toxic and non-irritant, although may cause contact dermatitis in hypersensitive individuals.

Jasmine
(Jasminum officinalis)

FAMILY: Oleaceae

DERIVATION: The essential oil must be extracted by enfleurage, resulting in an extremely costly oil.

ORIGINS/HISTORY: Jasmine's aroma has been so popular with gardeners that there are now around 40 different varieties cultivated in Britain, although it came originally from north west Asia and China. In India, it is sacred to the god Vishnu, and legend has it that Cleopatra used it to seduce Anthony.

THERAPEUTIC APPLICATIONS/PROPERTIES: Because Jasmine is so costly, it is not much used in home aromatherapy, but like all essential oils it does have therapeutic uses. Its heady, uplifting scent has been used since antiquity as a mood-enhancing agent, and as such it is useful in the treatment of stress-related illnesses. It also has smoothing, softening and balancing effects on skin and is a valuable component in skin care preparations. It also seems to have a regulating effect on the menstrual cycle, and has been successfully used in the alleviation of throat problems, coughs and catarrh. However, as there are many less expensive oils that will perform these functions, Jasmine's main use is as a fragrance ingredient in many high class perfumes.

OTHER USES: One of the mainstays of the perfume industry. Perfume ingredient in toiletries, soaps etc. Widely used in commercially-prepared foods and drinks.

SAFETY PRECAUTIONS/CONTRAINDICATIONS: Non-toxic and non-irritant, although has occasionally cased allergic reaction in sensitive individuals.

Juniper Berry
(Juniperus communis)

FAMILY: Cupressaceae

DERIVATION: The essential oil is distilled from the berries.

ORIGINS/HISTORY: Juniper is native to and widely distributed throughout the northern hemisphere. It has been valued as a herb with magical properties since the middle ages, when it was believed to keep witches at bay. The English herbalist Culpeper noted its diuretic properties in the 17th century, and used it to treat coughs and shortness of breath. More recently, French army nurses used burning juniper as an air disinfectant in the field hospitals of World War II.

THERAPEUTIC APPLICATIONS/PROPERTIES: Juniper seems to be beneficial to the digestive system , the female reproductive system and the menstrual cycle. It also helps regulate problem skin and is favoured by therapists in the treatment of acne, eczema, dermatitis and haemorrhoids. It helps disperse uric acid build-up and is therefore useful in the treatment of gout and other joint problems. It is a good stress-reliever, especially when used in the bath, and has a mild diuretic action which indicates its use in cystitis. Juniper also acts as an appetite stimulant, and is often used to get rid of intestinal parasites.

OTHER USES: Juniper is the main flavour ingredient in gin. Used in veterinary preparations for the prevention of infestation. A popular spicy aroma used in perfumes and aftershaves.

SAFETY PRECAUTIONS/CONTRAINDICATIONS: Juniper stimulates uterine contractions, therefore should not be used in pregnancy. It should also be avoided by those with kidney disease. Otherwise, Juniper is generally non-toxic but may be slightly irritant.

Lavender
(Lavandula vera or L. officinalis)

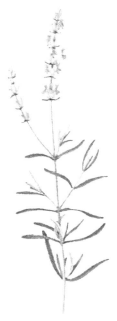

FAMILY: Lamiaceae (*Labiateae*)

DERIVATION: The essential oil is obtained by steam distillation from the flowers of the plant.

ORIGINS/HISTORY: Lavender is indigenous to mountainous regions of the western Mediterranean and widely cultivated in Britain. In days gone by it was used as a condiment and flavouring, and as a furniture polish. It has also been used for centuries to scent linen and as a toilet water.

THERAPEUTIC APPLICATIONS/PROPERTIES: Lavender is an appetite stimulant, a tonic and an antispasmodic. It is particularly effective in the treatment of minor burns and scalds, wounds, sores and varicose ulcers, and is generally one of the most versatile and widely used oils for healing. It also has a strong antiseptic effect and is employed in many cosmetic preparations and as an insect repellent. It is also used in the treatment of muscular aches and pains, respiratory problems, influenza, digestive problems, and genito-urinary problems such as cystitis and dysmenorrhoea. Its soothing and relaxing effect is recommended for depression, headaches and pre-menstrual tension.

OTHER USES: Antiseptic and fragrance ingredient in pharmaceutical preparations. Used in all kinds of perfumes, household cleaners, soaps and toiletries.

SAFETY PRECAUTIONS/CONTRAINDICATIONS: Lavender is an extremely safe oil and can even be applied undiluted to the skin.

Lemon
(Citrus limonium)

FAMILY: Rutaceae

DERIVATION: The oil is obtained by expression of the skin of the mature fruit.

ORIGINS / HISTORY: Lemons were indigenous to south east Asia, but are now widely cultivated throughout the Mediterranean countries. The Romans gave their pregnant women lemon cordials to prevent morning sickness—in fact the oil is still used to alleviate nausea and as an appetite stimulant. In some early Christian art, it is lemon rather than apple which Eve plucked from the tree of knowledge and ate, resulting in her expulsion from the garden of Eden with Adam.

THERAPEUTIC APPLICATIONS / PROPERTIES: As a massage oil lemon can have a very stimulating effect on the circulation, and seems to have the ability to stimulate the body's own immune system. Therefore, it is frequently used to treat circulatory problems and respiratory ailments such as asthma, bronchitis and catarrh. As a digestive aid, lemon can have a calming effect on dyspepsia. As a natural cosmetic, lemon has an astringent and toning effect, and also acts as a natural deodorant.

OTHER USES: Used as a flavouring in a variety of pharmaceutical preparations such as lozenge and cough medicines. A fragrance ingredient in perfumes, soaps, toiletries and household cleaners.

SAFETY PRECAUTIONS / CONTRAINDICATIONS: Lemon is generally very safe, but should be applied in moderation and in the correct dilution to the skin, and should not be used prior to exposure to sunlight.

Lemongrass
(Cymbopogon citratus)

FAMILY: Poaceae (*Gramineae*)

DERIVATION: The oil is obtained by steam distillation from the leaves of the grass.

ORIGINS/HISTORY: Lemongrass is indigenous to Asia (particularly to Sri Lanka), Brazil and parts of South Africa. It has been used in traditional Indian medicine for centuries, primarily for treating fever and infectious disease. It has an extremely strong odour which is often intensely disliked.

THERAPEUTIC APPLICATIONS/PROPERTIES: Combined with neroli in a massage oil, lemongrass brings relief to muscular aches and pains. It is also credited with having a sedative effect on the central nervous system, inducing a deep sense of relaxation when used in the bath. Lemongrass has an extremely strong bactericidal and fungicidal effect which indicates its use in a variety of infections such as athlete's foot and thrush. It is also helpful in digestive disturbances such as colitis and indigestion, especially where stress or anxiety are a predisposing factor.

OTHER USES: Used as a fragrance ingredient in soaps, household cleaners and perfumes. A flavouring ingredient of foods and drinks.

SAFETY PRECAUTIONS/CONTRAINDICATIONS: Generally non-toxic, but occasionally dermatitis has been reported in sensitive individuals. Use under the guidance of a trained aromatherapist.

Mandarin
(Citrus nobilis, C. reticulata)

FAMILY: Rutaceae

DERIVATION: The oil is expressed from the outer peel of the fruit.

ORIGINS / HISTORY: Mandarin is native to southern China and was a traditional gift to Chinese mandarins—hence the name. The name tangerine was given to the fruit by the Americans in the 1840s upon its introduction to the country. In France it has long been regarded as the oil of choice in the treatment of liver or digestive problems in the elderly and for children's ailments.

THERAPEUTIC APPLICATIONS / PROPERTIES: Mandarin is still a popular oil in the treatment of digestive weaknesses and liver disturbances and is especially preferred for children and the elderly on account of its gentle nature. For stress, anxiety, insomnia and nervousness, its use is recommended in conjunction with other citrus oils. Like neroli, it is also a wonderful skin tonic, particularly for acne and oily skins. It is also indicated in the treatment of fluid retention.

OTHER USES: Mandarin's gentle aroma is popular in soaps, perfumes and cosmetic preparations. It is used to flavour many foods, particularly sweets. Also used to flavour liqueurs and soft drinks.

SAFETY PRECAUTIONS / CONTRAINDICATIONS: Generally very safe, although there may be a tendency towards phototoxicity. Therefore, its use on the skin is not recommended prior to exposure to sunlight.

Marjoram (Sweet)

(*Origanum marjorama*)

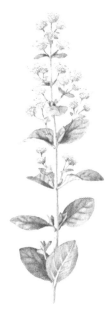

FAMILY: Lamiaceae (*Labiatae*)

DERIVATION: The essential oil is extracted by steam distillation from the dried leaves and flowering tops.

ORIGINS/HISTORY: Marjoram is native to Portugal where it is perennial, but must usually be grown annually in cooler climes. Historically, it was woven into wreaths for newlyweds to wear for luck. Greek physicians used it as an antidote to poison and snakebites, and the Romans for giddiness and upset stomachs.

THERAPEUTIC APPLICATIONS/PROPERTIES: Marjoram can be extremely effective in reducing the pain and swelling of muscular damage, bruises and sprains, and arthritis. It has an extremely hypnotic effect, which is useful in inducing sleep and calming emotions, especially when used in the bath. It can also be effective in menstrual problems. Marjoram is also a popular treatment for colds and coughs, bronchitis and asthma, and has a carminative and antispasmodic action on colic, constipation and flatulence.

OTHER USES: Detergents, cosmetics, soaps and perfumes. Many culinary uses. Used to flavour some alcoholic beverages.

SAFETY PRECAUTIONS/CONTRAINDICATIONS: Should be avoided by pregnant women as it has a strong emmenagogic effect. Not to be confused with Spanish Marjoram (*Thymus masttichina*), which is often sold commercially as 'Marjoram'.

Melissa True
(Melissa officinalis)

FAMILY: Lamiaceae (*Labiatae*)

DERIVATION: Derived from the leaves and flowers by steam distillation, it is rarely stocked commercially as it is expensive to produce, but is often sold as a blend without the same properties.

ORIGINS/HISTORY: Also known as lemon balm or sweet balm, it is one of the earliest herbs to have been used medicinally. Originally native to the Mediterranean, it is now grown throughout Europe.

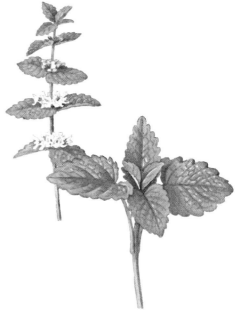

THERAPEUTIC APPLICATIONS/PROPERTIES: Melissa is used in the treatment of respiratory disorders, nausea, indigestion and skin disorders. It is said to regulate menstruation and fertility, and is helpful in the treatment of anxiety and depression because of its revitalising properties. It also relieves and aids healing of wasp and bee stings. The British Pharmacopoeia recommends it for flatulent dyspepsia, neurasthenia and depressive illness.

OTHER USES: Perfumes, soups, cosmetics and toiletries. Many culinary uses: also used by the food and pharmaceutical industries.

SAFETY PRECAUTIONS/CONTRAINDICATIONS: Has caused occasional sensitization and dermal irritations and is therefore best used in low concentrations. Rarely stocked commercially, most melissa are blends and should be labelled so.

Myrrh
(Commiphora myrrha)

FAMILY: Burseraceae

DERIVATION: The oil is derived from solvent extraction of the crude myrrh, which seeps from the trunk of the tree.

ORIGINS/HISTORY: Myrrh is a native of north east Africa and the Yemen, Somalia and Ethiopia. It was highly prized in the ancient world, and has been used since time immemorial as an ingredient in perfumes and incense, in the holy oil of the Jews and by the Egyptians in their embalming Kyphi. The Greeks used myrrh to disinfect wounds and promote healing, and also favoured it for skin complaints. Mention has been made of medicinal use of myrrh in records dating back 3700 years.

THERAPEUTIC APPLICATIONS/PROPERTIES: Myrrh has a stimulant effect on the mucous membranes and is therefore a useful expectorant and is helpful in the treatment of catarrh. It is still used in Chinese medicine to treat menstrual disturbances and complaints, haemorrhoids and sores. It is also indicated for dental problems—indeed it is a popular ingredient for toothpaste—and is an effective antiseptic gargle for throat infections. It has long been known as an appetite stimulant and is a valuable ingredient in beauty treatments for mature skin.

OTHER USES: Toothpastes, gargles and mouthwashes. Soups, cosmetics, detergents and perfumes. Food and drink flavouring agent.

SAFETY PRECAUTIONS/CONTRAINDICATIONS: Myrrh has an emmenagogic action, therefore should not be used by pregnant women.

Neroli
(Citrus aurantium var. amara)

FAMILY: Rutaceae

DERIVATION: Derived from steam or solvent distillation from the freshly picked flowers.

ORIGINS/HISTORY: Originally a native of the Far East, the tree now grows throughout the Mediterranean. Neroli is thought to be named after the 16th-century Italian princess Neroli, who scented her rooms and gowns with it. Orange flowers were traditionally included in wedding flower arrangement, as the soothing scent was said to be necessary to relax the newlyweds before they withdrew to the marriage bed.

THERAPEUTIC APPLICATIONS/PROPERTIES: Neroli is an extremely expensive oil to produce because of the volume of flowers required, but it is very much in demand in perfumery because of its wonderful aroma. This is frequently harnessed in massage oil because of its power to uplift, calm and relax. It is also believed to have qualities which are extremely beneficial to the skin, and is widely used to preserve skin elasticity, to prevent stretch marks and scarring, to reduce thread veins and as an aid for dry, sensitive skin. Neroli's stress-relieving qualities indicate its use in a wide variety of stress-related complaints, ranging from colitis and diarrhoea to palpitations, insomnia and PMT.

OTHER USES: High class, expensive perfumes, toilet waters and eau-de-cologne. Very occasionally a flavour ingredient in foodstuffs.

SAFETY PRECAUTIONS/CONTRAINDICATIONS: None.

Nutmeg
(*Myristica fragraus*)

FAMILY: Myristicaceae

ORIGINS/HISTORY: Native to the Middle East and West Indies, although that grown in the 'East Indies' is usually considered superior. Nutmeg has been used in the treatment of digestive and kidney complaints for centuries. Malaysians still use it as a uterine tonic, and a little grated nutmeg mixed with lard constitutes a centuries-old remedy for piles.

DERIVATION: Nutmeg oil can be extracted by steam or water distillation from either the dried seed or husk (mace).

THERAPEUTIC APPLICATIONS/PROPERTIES: Nutmeg is recommended in the British Herbal Pharmacopoeia for a variety of digestive complaints such as dysentery, nausea, dyspepsia, flatulence and diarrhoea. It can be applied locally for rheumatism. Its warming effects are particularly welcome in the winter, and it has strong, stimulant properties which lend it to the treatment of poor circulation, poor appetite and menstrual irregularities.

OTHER USES: A very popular flavouring agent in the pharmaceutical and food industries. Used widely in detergents, soaps, lotions and perfumes—particularly men's fragrances.

SAFETY PRECAUTIONS/CONTRAINDICATIONS: Not to be used in high doses or for extended periods of time, as essential oil of nutmeg can induce hallucinations and hypnosis. Avoid during pregnancy. Nutmeg should always be well diluted, even for bathing purposes as it can cause skin irritation.

> NUTMEG OIL CAN BE DANGEROUS AND SHOULD BE USED ONLY UNDER THE
> SUPERVISION OF A TRAINED AROMATHERAPIST.

Orange (Sweet)
(*Citrus sinensis*)

FAMILY: Rutaceae

DERIVATION: Essential oil is obtained by cold expression or steam distillation of the ripe peel of the fruit.

ORIGINS / HISTORY: Sweet Orange is originally a native of China but is now extensively cultivated, being particularly popular in Florida and California and in the Mediterranean. Traditional Chinese medical practitioners have used dried sweet orange peel to treat a variety of ailments including respiratory problems, anorexia and malignant breast lesions.

THERAPEUTIC APPLICATIONS / PROPERTIES: Sweet orange essential oil is very useful in the treatment of respiratory infections such as colds, bronchitis and influenza, and is thought to increase bronchial secretions. It can also help oily and dull complexions when used as part of a skin care routine. Having similar stress-relieving qualities to neroli, it is also helpful in the alleviation of stress-related complaints. As a gentle aid to digestion, it is often used to ease dyspepsia and constipation.

OTHER USES: Pharmaceutical flavouring. Detergents, soaps, cosmetics and perfumes, especially eau-de-cologne. Frequently used as a flavouring in the food manufacturing industry.

SAFETY PRECAUTIONS / CONTRAINDICATIONS: Generally safe, but distilled essential oil of orange is photo toxic and should not be applied to the skin prior to exposure to sunlight.

Parsley
(Carum petroselinum)

FAMILY: Apiaceae (*Umbelliferae*)

ORIGINS/HISTORY: Parsley is native to the Mediterranean, and was introduced to the British Isles in the 16th century. It has become completely naturalised in some parts of England and Scotland. The Ancient Greeks crowned the victors of the Isthmia games with crowns of parsley and adorned the tombs of the dead with parsley wreaths.

THERAPEUTIC APPLICATIONS/PROPERTIES: Parsley has a diuretic and emmenagogic effect which makes it useful for menstrual problems. It also has the power to reduce fever and has a soothing effect on colic, flatulence and indigestion. It is used for treating bladder and kidney problems, and is also indicated in the treatment of arthritis, rheumatism and sciatica, cystitis and urinary tract infections.

OTHER USES: Parsley is frequently included in digestive remedies. Fragrance ingredient in household cleaners, cosmetics, perfumes and colognes, particularly fragrances for men. Used extensively in cookery and in the food industry.

SAFETY PRECAUTIONS/CONTRAINDICATIONS: Oil of parsley is moderately toxic, therefore it is wise to use it in moderation, and to avoid it completely in pregnancy.

PARSLEY OIL CAN BE DANGEROUS AND SHOULD BE USED ONLY UNDER THE SUPERVISION OF A TRAINED AROMATHERAPIST.

Patchouli
(Pogostemon patchouli)

FAMILY: Lamiaceae (*Labiatae*)

DERIVATION: Essential oil is extracted by steam distillation from the seed and the herb.

ORIGINS/HISTORY: Patchouli is native to Bengal, India, the West Indies and Paraguay. It has a very distinctive and well-known aroma which is either loved or hated and has the unusual quality of improving with age. Victorians used it to scent Indian ink, and as a moth repellent. In China, the herb is used medicinally to treat a variety of ailments.

THERAPEUTIC APPLICATIONS/PROPERTIES: Patchouli possesses a soothing, calming earthy scent. It is a good antiseptic with anti-inflammatory properties, which makes it a sensible choice in the treatment of minor burns. Patchouli has also been credited with aphrodisiac powers, and is excellent for relieving a variety of skin disorders including acne, athlete's foot, eczema and dry and cracked skin. It is also used for treating poisonous snakebites in Japan and Malaysia.

OTHER USES: Insect repellent. Masking agents—covers unpleasant smells. Used as a fixative in oriental perfumes and soaps.

SAFETY PRECAUTIONS/CONTRAINDICATIONS: None.

Peppermint
(Mentha piperita)

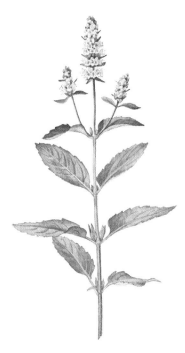

FAMILY: Lamiaceae (*Labiatae*)

DERIVATION: The essential oil is extracted from the flowering herb by steam distillation.

ORIGINS/HISTORY: Found throughout Europe. The Greeks and Romans crowned themselves with peppermint at feasts and adorned their tables with it. Two species were used by the ancient Greek physicians, but it is unclear as to whether or not this is exactly the same peppermint used today. (Peppermint came into general use in England in the mid 18th century). A form of peppermint has been discovered in Egyptian tombs dating as far back as 1000BC.

THERAPEUTIC APPLICATIONS/PROPERTIES: Peppermint has a marked anti-spasmodic effect and is useful in the treatment of abdominal cramps and digestive upsets. Oil of peppermint allays sickness and nausea, and its invigorating aroma can often alleviate respiratory problems and the symptoms of colds and flu. It is an extremely gentle inhalation for asthma, and very effective in the relief of morning sickness.

OTHER USES: Commercial food flavouring. Pharmaceutical cold and digestive preparations. Flavouring element in dental preparation. Perfumes, colognes.

SAFETY PRECAUTIONS/CONTRAINDICATIONS: Possibly irritant to sensitive skin—use in moderation always.

Petitgrain
(Citrus aurantium var. amara)

FAMILY: Rutaceae

DERIVATION: The oil is distilled from the leaves and the twigs.

ORIGINS / HISTORY: Native to China and India, although nowadays France produces the best quality oil. The name originally came from the tiny unripe fruits from which the oil was extracted.

THERAPEUTIC APPLICATIONS / PROPERTIES: Petitgrain can be used as a mild antidepressant substitute for neroli, and is effective in the alleviation of anxiety and insomnia. It is also valuable in skin care, having a balancing and toning effect on greasy skin conditions. In the digestive system, it reduces the symptoms of dyspepsia and flatulence.

OTHER USES: Used for its fragrance in soaps, household cleaners, perfumes and cosmetics. It is a popular flavouring ingredient.

SAFETY PRECAUTIONS / CONTRAINDICATIONS: None.

Pine

(Over 100 varieties—the most commonly used is *Pinus sylvestris*)

FAMILY: Pinaceae

DERIVATION: The oil is obtained by dry distillation from the needles.

ORIGINS/HISTORY: Pine was originally a native of Eurasia, but is now widely cultivated. Avicenna, the ancient Arab physician, recommended the use of pine oil in poultices and inhalations for pneumonia. The needles were traditionally used by American Indians as a prophylactic against scurvy and also to stuff mattresses as a lice and flea repellent.

THERAPEUTIC APPLICATIONS/PROPERTIES: Pine has a strong antiseptic quality, valued for its effectiveness in treating respiratory conditions and relieving asthma, blocked sinuses and catarrh when used as an inhalation. Its stimulating effect also makes it a good choice as a warming massage oil for muscular pains and strains. It has a multitude of other applications: for cuts and sores, arthritis and rheumatism, cystitis and urinary tract infections, fatigue, stress, anxiety and neuralgia.

OTHER USES: Veterinary antiseptic sprays, disinfectants, fragrance ingredient in perfumes, household cleaners, soaps and toiletries.

SAFETY PRECAUTIONS/CONTRAINDICATIONS: Those with a tendency towards sensitive skin should avoid bathing in pine oil.

PINE OIL SHOULD ONLY BE USED BY A TRAINED AROMATHERAPIST AND IS UNSAFE FOR HOME USE.

Rose
(Rosa centifola, r. damascena)

FAMILY: Rosaceae

DERIVATION: Obtained by steam distillation or solvent extraction from the fresh petals.

ORIGINS/HISTORY: Rose is believed to be native to the Orient, now cultivated throughout the world. Culpeper recommended oil of roses to cool hot inflammations or swellings. The rose has been a symbol of romance and love for many centuries.

THERAPEUTIC APPLICATIONS/PROPERTIES: A supremely feminine and deeply sensual aroma which is the mainstay of the perfume industry. Rose oil has a wonderful anti-depressant effect which may be harnessed in body and face massages, baths or vaporisers to treat anxiety, stress and depression. It also has a gentle balancing effect on gynaecological disorders, and has an aphrodisiac effect.

OTHER USES: The rose is a mainstay of the perfume industry. Cosmetics and toiletries. Occasionally used as a flavouring.

SAFETY PRECAUTIONS/CONTRAINDICATIONS: None.

Rosemary
(Rosemarinus officinalis)

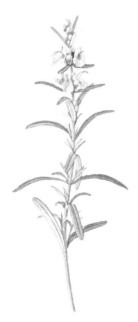

FAMILY: Lamiaceae (*Labiatae*)

DERIVATION: The oil is extracted by steam distillation from the flowering tops of the plant.

ORIGINS/HISTORY: Rosemary was originally native to the Mediterranean, and is now cultivated throughout the world. The ancients were well acquainted with this herb, which had a reputation for enhancing the memory. It was also used at weddings and was worn as a symbol of fidelity for lovers. Rosemary has long been regarded as an elixir of youth.

THERAPEUTIC APPLICATIONS/PROPERTIES: Rosemary has a wide application and is effective in the treatment of numerous complaints. Possessing a powerful aroma, Rosemary is favoured as a decongestant in inhalation and an invigorating muscle-strengthening massage oil. Skin and hair problems can respond well to Rosemary, and gargling in it will freshen the breath. Above all, Rosemary seems to possess remarkable memory and concentration-enhancing properties. Other therapeutic uses are in digestive disorders, hypercholesterolaemia, headaches and stress.

OTHER USES: Fragrance ingredient in soaps, perfumes and household cleaners. Used as a flavouring in food production. A natural anti-oxidant.

SAFETY PRECAUTIONS/CONTRAINDICATIONS: Avoid during pregnancy. Should not be used by epileptics.

Sage
(*Salvia officinalis*)

FAMILY: Lamiaceae (*Labiatae*)

DERIVATION: The leaves are best dried naturally, then the oil is extracted by steam distillation.

ORIGINS / HISTORY: Native to the northern shores of the Mediterranean. Sage was held in high esteem in classical times and throughout the Middle Ages. In the Jura district of France, the herb is believed to have the power of healing and lessening grief, as is borne out by the old French saying: 'Sage helps the nerves and by its powerful might Palsy is cured and fever put to flight.'

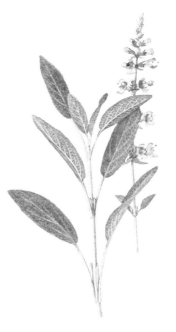

THERAPEUTIC APPLICATIONS / PROPERTIES: Sage has an expectorant effect when used in inhalations, and its astringent and cooling properties make it a popular choice as a tonic, an appetite stimulant and as a fever reducer. Its antiseptic effects are beneficial to sore throats and mouth problems if used in a gargle or mouthwash. Sage can also be burnt in sick rooms to purify the air. It is also helpful in rheumatism and arthritis, bronchitis and catarrh, sprains, bruises and headaches.

OTHER USES: Used in pharmaceutical preparations. Fragrance ingredient for perfumes, household cleaners, toiletries. Flavouring in the food industry.

SAFETY PRECAUTIONS / CONTRAINDICATIONS: Avoid during pregnancy and in epilepsy. Sage is toxic if ingested and is best substituted with Spanish sage or clary sage for home use.

Sandalwood
(Santalum album)

FAMILY: Santalaceae

DERIVATION: The essential oil is obtained by steam distillation from the wood of the sandalwood tree.

ORIGINS/HISTORY: Sandalwood is native to India where it formed part of the Ayurvedic tradition. It was traditionally used in the funeral rites and embalming of Singhalese princes, and still has an important ceremonial role in Hindu marriages. According to tradition, Burmese women sprinkle sandalwood oil mixed with rosewater on passers-by at New Year in order to cleanse them of the year's sins.

THERAPEUTIC APPLICATIONS/PROPERTIES: Its preservative powers are often employed to lengthen the life of creams and potions. Sandalwood is a wonderful facial oil, with a soothing emollient effect on dry or sensitive skin. It cleanses, softens and helps to heal problem skin. This oil also has a powerful relaxing effect, and can alleviate upset stomachs, especially where nervous tension or stress has been a causative factor. Sandalwood also seems to have a powerful antiseptic effect which is particularly useful in the treatment of cystitis and urinary tract infections. It is also favoured for menstrual problems, as a sedative and for catarrh.

Other Uses: Widely used as a fragrance and a fixative in perfumes. Used as a flavouring in food production.

SAFETY PRECAUTIONS/CONTRAINDICATIONS: None.

Tea Tree
(Melaleuca alternifolia)

FAMILY: Myrtaceae

DERIVATION: The oil is extracted by steam or water distillation from the leaves and twigs of the tree.

ORIGINS/HISTORY: Native to the Antipodes. Early European settlers in Australia and New Zealand used the aromatic leaves of this tree to make tea, hence the name 'tea tree'. Captain Cook also found it invaluable in overcoming scurvy in his sailors. However, the aborigines were already aware if its healing properties, using the leaves in poultices to treat wounds.

THERAPEUTIC APPLICATIONS/PROPERTIES: Tea tree is strongly disinfectant, antibacterial, anti-fungal, anti-viral and antiseptic—all qualities which make tea tree an invaluable weapon in the treatment of a multitude of infections. Similarly, tea tree also seems to offer a boost to the body's own immune system whenever threat of infection occurs. Tea tree should be considered when treating any of the following problems: colds, influenza, bronchitis and asthma, warts and verrucas, burns and inflammation, thrush and similar fungal infections, mild shock and hysteria.

OTHER USES: A fragrance and disinfectant ingredient in many toiletries and household cleaning products. Pharmaceutical preparations. Fragrance ingredient in perfumes and aftershaves.

SAFETY PRECAUTIONS/CONTRAINDICATIONS: Generally very safe, but may cause sensitisation in some people.

Thyme (Sweet)
(*Thymus vulgaris*)

FAMILY: Lamiaceae (*Labiatae*)

DERIVATION: The oil is obtained by steam distillation from the plant's flowering tops.

ORIGINS/HISTORY: In its wild form, thyme was originally native to Spain and other countries bordering the Mediterranean, and commonly cultivated in this country by the mid 16th century. Thyme has a long history as a medicinal herb, and was used by the Egyptians in embalming. The ancient Greeks had great belief in its disease-combating powers and used it as a fumigation.

THERAPEUTIC APPLICATIONS/PROPERTIES: Thyme is a strong antiseptic, perhaps the strongest of any oil, and is also a powerful stimulant to the appetite, the immune system, and the central nervous system. Respiratory infections, coughs and asthma all seem to respond well to thyme oil, especially if used in inhalations and gargles. (N.B. Gargles must not be swallowed) and care must be taken to use the thyme in low dilutions. Its use is indicated in a wide variety of fungal, bacterial and viral infections, in the treatment of wounds and sores and as an aid to the immune system.

OTHER USES: A popular addition to mouthwashes, gargles, cough preparations and toothpastes. Used in the food and drink industry as a flavouring.

SAFETY PRECAUTIONS/CONTRAINDICATIONS: Not to be applied undiluted to the skin or used during pregnancy, or on children's skin. Always dilute prior to use in the bath, in fact, generally best used in low concentrations.

> THERE ARE SEVERAL TYPES OF THYME, SOME OF WHICH CAN BE DANGEROUS.
> ONLY SWEET THYME IS SAFE FOR HOME USE.

Ylang Ylang
(Cananga odorata var. genuina)

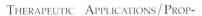

FAMILY: Annonaceae

DERIVATION: The oil is obtained by steam distillation from the flowers.

ORIGINS / HISTORY: Ylang Ylang is native to Indonesia, the Philippines, Madagascar and Java. Indonesian newlyweds traditionally have their marriage beds spread with Ylang Ylang flowers.

THERAPEUTIC APPLICATIONS / PROPERTIES: Like most essential oils Ylang Ylang has a strong antiseptic effect, but it is best known for its euphoric and aphrodisiac properties. The nervous system can also benefit greatly from its relaxing powers, and its antidepressant powers can be harnessed to treat mild shock, anger and stress. It is used widely as an ingredient in skin care, having a wonderful tonic effect and gentle action. It can also be helpful in the regulation of high blood pressure and tachycardia (excessively fast heartbeat.)

OTHER USES: A wonderful fragrance for perfumes, soap, cosmetics. A flavour ingredient, used mainly in desserts and drinks.

SAFETY PRECAUTIONS / CONTRAINDICATIONS: Generally very safe, although sensitisation has been reported in a small number of cases. Used excessively, it can cause nausea or headache.

Massage

Contraindications

For most people, massage is a wonderfully relaxing experience, and has great therapeutic value, especially when used in conjunction with aromatic oils. However, there are some conditions for which massage is inadvisable, and if in doubt, it is always prudent to check with a medical practitioner prior to commencement.

Massage is not advised in the following conditions:

Heart Disease
Bone Fractures
Recent Scarring
Severe Bruising
Epilepsy
Haemorrhage
Area of contagious skin disease
Severe Sunburn
Extreme Hypertension or Hypotension
Uncontrolled Diabetes
On the Abdomen and Lower Back during Pregnancy
Open Wound
Undiagnosed Lumps
Nausea
Extreme Unexplained Tenderness

High Temperature
Osteoporosis
Varicose Veins
Cancer

Persistent, painful or chronic conditions should never be treated by aromatherapy without seeking medical advice. In the home, aromatherapy should only be used for minor complaints, minor first aid, and for stress relief and relaxation.

Types of Massage

The type of massage is generally a matter of personal preference of the masseur, and aromatherapists may favour more than one form.

Remedial Massage

This form of massage is used to treat specific muscular problems or injuries, rather than for relaxation. The techniques employed often involve deep tissue massage to promote circulation to the injured part, and can sometimes cause discomfort.

Swedish Massage

This form of massage was pioneered in the late 19th century by Per Henrik Ling. He analysed ancient massage techniques, and clarified their application. It is primarily used by beauty therapists today, but constitutes a useful 'all-over' massage technique which will stimulate the circulation and lymphatic drainage. This type of massage is very relaxing.

Mechanical Massage

This involves the use of percussors and gyrators, and are primarily used to conserve the energy of the therapist. However, they are not always suitable for aromatherapy, as many oils will have a corrosive effect on the rubber parts of the appliances in time.

Shiatsu

Shiatsu is an ancient Eastern technique which requires the therapist to apply pressure with his/her fingers, elbows, knees and feet. It works from the premise that all the energies the body flow along ancient lines known as meridians, and that these are prone to blockage. Shiatsu aims to restore the flow of energy by unblocking these lines using specific pressure points on the body. It is claimed that Shiatsu massage will rid the body of disease by restoring the natural flow of energy.

Reflexology

Reflexology is an art dating back to ancient times , and was used by the Egyptians as testified by paintings in the pyramids.

Reflexology uses 'zones' or 'reflex points' on the feet and hands which are meant to connect to various glands, organs or parts of the body. The technique aims to exert pressure upon congested area, ultimately clearing them and thus aiding the immune system. It is said to be particularly beneficial to the smooth operation of the lymph and endocrine glands.

Aromassage at Home

Before beginning an aromatherapy massage, there are a number of steps which should be taken in order for the subject of the massage to derive full benefit from the treatment.

1   It is important to take a brief history from the patient in order to be able to select the correct oils. This will involve an assessment of his/her emotional state as well as any physical complaints.

2   At least an hour should have elapsed since the last meal prior to receiving or giving a massage.

3   Make sure your clothing is loose and will not obstruct your movements.

4   Ensure that hands are clean and nails short.

5   Have some tissues ready, and make sure your oil is easily accessible.

6   Make sure your hands are warm before touching your subject.

The room should be warm so that your subject will be comfortable even though only partly dressed. Lighting should be subdued, and the telephone should be disconnected to avoid interruption. Perhaps music could be played softly in the background, but this is a matter of preference and convenience. It is a good idea to have a compatible essence evaporating in the room prior to commencement. The massage surface needs to be firm, therefore a normal sprung bed is unsuitable—rather pad the floor or use a futon or similar firm mattress.

First of all the subject may have a warm bath or shower in order that the pores are open and receptive to the essential oil. (This, however, is a matter of personal preference on the part of the therapist.) He/she should be positioned comfortably, and should be covered with towels, exposing only that area which is to be massaged at any one time in order to avoid embarrassment and cold. Hair should be tied out of the way.

Some Basic Massage Techniques

The following constitutes only a very basic guide to aromatherapy massage movements, and is no substitute for a comprehensive recognised aromamassage course. However, massage can be used to great benefit at home using the following simple movements and suggestions.

Effleurage

This is the most often used aromassage movement, and constitutes a simple, gentle stroking movement. (N.B. Deep pressure should never be used by an untrained person.) The strokes may be long or short, gentle or firm, but the whole hands should be used, always pushing the blood towards the heart thus promoting venus return. This stroke promotes muscle relaxation and soothes the nerve endings.

Petrissage

In petrissage, the flesh is rolled between the thumbs and fingers in a movement not unlike kneading dough. This technique is best used on the back and on fatty areas. The idea is to stimulate the circulation and lymphatic flow and thereby increase the rate of toxin expulsion.

Head massage

Put a little of the chosen essential oil in the fingertips and massage in circular movements over the scalp and temples.

Massage for tension headaches and migraine

Work from the base of the neck and scalp for a few moments, using effleurage strokes firmly, again with the chosen oil(s) on the fingertips

Massage for the neck

Working around the base of the neck and scalp, use small upward and out-ward circular movements. Move slowly upwards and downwards and around the sides of the neck, alternating firm and gentle movements.

Neck massage should be carried out with the patient in a supine position, or sitting on a chair with some support in front.

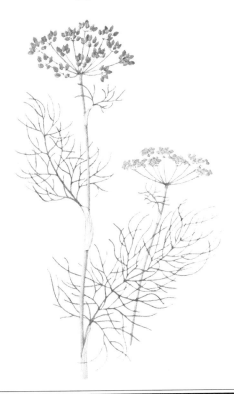

Fennel

Massage for the shoulders

Using anti-clockwise effleurage movements, stroke firmly from shoulders to neck.

Massage for the arms

Use effleurage and petrissage upwards in the direction of the armpit, concentrating on muscular and fatty areas. Avoid bony areas.

Massage for the back

Avoiding the vertebrae, use gentle or firm petrissage or effleurage technique. Stroke all the way from the lumbar to the shoulders, move the hands outwards across the shoulders and return slowly down the outer area of the back. Repeat this movement to induce deep relaxation.

Massage on the abdomen

Use only a gentle, clockwise effleurage stroke.

Massage for the legs

Legs should always be massaged in an upward direction. Avoid bony areas, and never massage varicose veins.

Massage for menstrual/gynaecological problems

Always use gentle effleurage movements and do not exert any pressure on the lower abdomen. Begin at the lower back and slide forwards and downwards across the hips. Repeat several times.

Massage for the feet

Work in the direction of toe to heel, using the fingers uppermost and the thumb under the foot.

Essential Oils & Common Ailments

* When employed incorrectly the oils marked * can have adverse effects and are normally recommended to be used under the guidance of a professional aromatherapist.

Stress Related Disorders

	Anxiety	Mild Shock	Depression	Mental fatigue
*Aniseed				
Basil	+	+		
*Bay				
Benzoin				
Bergamot	+		+	
Cajeput				
Cedarwood				
Chamomile		+	+	
*Cinnamon				
Clary Sage				+
*Clove				
Cypress				
Eucalyptus				+
Fennel (Sweet)				
Frankinsense				
Geranium	+		+	
Jasmine			+	
Juniper Berry				+
Lavender	+		+	
Lemon				
*Lemongrass				
Mandarin				
Marjoram (Sweet)	+			
Melissa	+	+		
Myyrh				
Neroli	+		+	
*Nutmeg				
Orange (Sweet)				
*Parsley				
Patchouli			+	
Peppermint		+		+
Petitgrain				
Pine				
Rose			+	
Rosemary		+	+	+
*Sage			+	
Sandalwood	+			
Tea Tree				
*Thyme				
Ylang Ylang				

Skin Complaints/Disorders

	Acne	Dry Skin	Eczema	Oily Skn	Psoriasis	Spots
*Aniseed						
Basil						
*Bay						
Benzoin						
Bergamot	+	+			+	
Cajeput						
Cedarwood	+					
Chamomile	+	+	+		+	
*Cinnamon						
Clary Sage						
*Clove						
Cypress	+			+		
Eucalyptus	+				+	
Fennel (Sweet)	+					
Frankinsense						
Geranium	+	+	+			
Jasmine		+				
Juniper Berry	+		+			
Lavender	+	+	+		+	+
Lemon	+			+		
*Lemongrass						
Mandarin						
Marjoram (Sweet)						
Melissa		+	+			
Myyrh	+					
Neroli		+				
*Nutmeg						
Orange (Sweet)						
*Parsley	+					
Patchouli	+	+				
Peppermint					+	
Petitgrain	+					
Pine						
Rose	+					
Rosemary	+					
*Sage						
Sandalwood	+	+				
Tea Tree	+			+		+
*Thyme						
Ylang Ylang		+				

Feminine/Gynaecological Disorders

	Amenorrhoea	C Dysmenorrhoea	Hot flushes	Mastitis	Period Pain	PMT
*Aniseed						
Basil						
*Bay						
Benzoin						
Bergamot						
Cajeput						
Cedarwood						
Chamomile	+		+	+		
*Cinnamon						
Clary Sage	+		+	+	+	
*Clove						
Cypress		+				
Eucalyptus						
Fennel (Sweet)	+					
Frankinsense						
Geranium	+	+		+		+
Jasmine			+			
Juniper Berry						
Lavender			+	+	+	+
Lemon						
*Lemongrass						
Mandarin						
Marjoram (Sweet)					+	
Melissa						
Myyrh						
Neroli			+			+
*Nutmeg						
Orange (Sweet)						
*Parsley						
Patchouli						
Peppermint						
Petitgrain			+			+
Pine						
Rose		+		+		+
Rosemary						
*Sage	+					
Sandalwood			+			
Tea Tree						
*Thyme						
Ylang Ylang			+			